Navigating Mental Health Challenges
with Grace and Resilience

Gail D. Jacob's

Contents

Introduction

In this book, we will explore the transformative power of self-compassion, and how it can help us navigate mental health challenges with grace and resilience. Through the pages of this book, you will learn about the science behind self-compassion, and how it can help you develop a kinder and more understanding relationship with yourself. You will also discover practical strategies for cultivating self-compassion in your daily life, and learn how to use this powerful tool to support your mental health and well-being.

Chapter 1

The Science Of Self Compassion

Self-compassion and self-esteem are two related but distinct concepts in the field of psychology.

Self-esteem refers to the overall evaluation or appraisal of oneself. It is a subjective assessment of one's worthiness, abilities, and achievements. High self-esteem is associated with positive emotions, confidence, and a sense of mastery, while low self-esteem is linked to negative emotions, self-doubt, and feelings of inferiority.

On the other hand, self-compassion refers to treating oneself with kindness, care, and understanding when faced with personal shortcomings, failures, or difficult emotions. It involves acknowledging one's pain or suffering without judgment and responding with warmth and support. Self-compassion emphasizes the importance of being kind to oneself, rather than focusing solely on self-evaluation and comparison with others.

The science behind self-compassion suggests that it has numerous benefits for mental health and well-being. Research has shown that self-compassion is associated with lower levels of anxiety, depression, and stress, as well as higher levels of happiness, life satisfaction, and resilience. Additionally, self-compassionate individuals are less likely to engage in self-criticism and more likely to seek help when needed.

One of the main differences between self-compassion and self-esteem is that self-esteem can be fragile and easily disrupted by setbacks or criticism, while self-compassion is more stable and resilient. Self-compassion is also more focused on internal sources of validation and self-worth, while self-esteem is often linked to external validation and comparison with others.

Another important difference is that self-compassion is more inclusive and unconditional than self-esteem. While self-esteem is often contingent on meeting certain standards or achieving specific goals, self-compassion is available to everyone, regardless of their achievements or shortcomings. This makes self-compassion a more accessible and supportive approach to self-care and self-improvement.

While self-esteem and self-compassion are both important concepts in psychology, self-compassion offers a more flexible, inclusive, and supportive approach to self-care and personal growth. Practicing self-compassion can help individuals cultivate a more resilient and positive sense of self, even in the face of setbacks and difficulties.

The Three (3) Components Of Self Compassion

Self-compassion is a concept that involves treating oneself with the same kindness, care, and concern that one would offer to a good friend who is going through a difficult time. It consists of three main components, which are:

1. Self-kindness: Self-kindness is the first component of self-compassion. It involves being

gentle and understanding towards oneself, rather than being critical or harsh. It means treating oneself with warmth, support, and patience when faced with challenges or difficulties.

2. Common humanity: The second component of self-compassion is common humanity. This component emphasizes that suffering and difficulties are a part of the human experience, and that no one is perfect or immune to them. It helps individuals realize that they are

not alone in their struggles and that others also experience similar challenges.

3. Mindfulness: The third component of self-compassion is mindfulness. It involves being aware of and acknowledging one's thoughts and feelings without judgment or avoidance. Mindfulness allows individuals to observe their experiences and emotions without getting caught up in them, helping them develop a greater sense of self-awareness and understanding. It allows

individuals to approach their struggles with greater clarity and acceptance, which can lead to greater resilience and growth.

Together, these three components of self-compassion can help individuals cultivate a kinder, more supportive, and less judgmental relationship with themselves, which can lead to greater emotional well-being and resilience in the face of life's challenges.

The Benefits Of Self-compassion

Self-compassion has been shown to have numerous benefits for mental health and well-being.

One of the primary benefits of self-compassion is that it can help individuals navigate mental health challenges with greater ease and resilience. When individuals are facing difficult emotions or experiences, self-compassion allows them to acknowledge their pain without judgment or self-blame. This can help to reduce feelings of shame and isolation, which are often associated with mental health issues. Instead of feeling overwhelmed or helpless, individuals can use self-compassion to develop a sense of inner strength and resourcefulness, which can help them to cope with difficult situations.

Self-compassion has also been shown to improve mood and decrease symptoms of depression and anxiety. When individuals practice self-compassion, they are less likely to engage in negative self-talk and rumination, which are common in individuals with depression and anxiety. Instead, self-compassionate individuals tend to be more accepting of their emotions and experiences, which can help to reduce feelings of distress and improve overall mental health.

In addition to improving mental health, self-compassion has also been linked to better physical health outcomes. Studies have shown that individuals who practice self-compassion have lower levels of stress and inflammation, which are both risk factors for numerous health problems. By reducing stress and inflammation, self-compassion can help to improve overall physical health and well-being.

Overall, self-compassion is a powerful tool for improving mental health and navigating mental health challenges with greater ease and resilience. By treating oneself with kindness, concern, and understanding, individuals can cultivate a sense of inner strength and resourcefulness that can help them to cope with difficult situations and improve their overall well-being.

Chapter 2

Practical strategies for cultivating self compassion in your everyday life.

Here are some practical strategies for cultivating self-compassion in our everyday life:

1. Mindfulness: Practice mindfulness by focusing on the present moment and being aware of your thoughts and feelings. Mindfulness helps you to observe your thoughts and emotions without judgment, which can

help you respond to yourself with greater compassion.

2. Self-talk: Be kind to yourself in your self-talk. Avoid using negative self-talk and instead focus on positive affirmations that reinforce your self-worth and positive qualities.

3. Self-care: Engage in self-care activities that help you feel good about yourself. This could include taking a relaxing bath, going for a walk in nature, or treating yourself to something you enjoy.

4. Acceptance: Accept yourself as you are, including your flaws and imperfections. Recognize that everyone makes mistakes and has weaknesses, and that this is a normal part of being human.

5. Forgiveness: Forgive yourself for any mistakes or shortcomings. Practice letting go of negative self-judgment and focus on learning and growing from your experiences.

6. Gratitude: Practice gratitude by focusing on the positive aspects of your life. Expressing gratitude for the things you have can help you feel more positive and less critical of yourself.

7. Connection: Connect with others who support and encourage you. Surrounding yourself with positive, supportive people can help you cultivate self-compassion and improve your self-esteem.

Remember, self-compassion is a skill that can be developed over time with practice. Start by choosing one or two strategies that resonate with you and make them a regular part of your everyday life. Over time, you may find that your self-compassion grows stronger and becomes a natural part of your way of being.

Self Compassion, Empathy, Mindfulness.

Practicing self-kindness, developing a sense of common humanity, and cultivating mindfulness are all important aspects of personal growth and well-being. Here are some practical ways to integrate these practices into your daily life:

Self-Kindness:
a. Practice self-compassion: Be kind and understanding to yourself, especially in moments of failure or

disappointment. Treat yourself as you would a good friend.

b. Practice self-care: Take care of yourself physically, emotionally, and mentally. Make sure you get enough sleep, eat healthily, exercise regularly, and take breaks when you need them.

c. Identify your strengths and accomplishments: Celebrate your successes, even small ones, and recognize your strengths and talents.

d. Avoid self-criticism: Be mindful of negative self-talk and avoid harsh self-criticism. Instead, focus on constructive feedback and positive self-talk.

Common Humanity:
a. Practice empathy: Try to understand others' perspectives and experiences, even if you don't agree with them.

b. Connect with others: Engage in social activities and build positive relationships with people around you.

c. Volunteer: Helping others can create a sense of connection and shared humanity.

d. Avoid comparison: Recognize that everyone has their own struggles and challenges, and avoid comparing yourself to others.

Mindfulness:

a. Practice meditation: Set aside a few minutes each day to meditate, focus on your breath, and be present in the moment.

b. Stay present: Pay attention to your thoughts, feelings, and physical sensations throughout the day.

c. Slow down: Take breaks throughout the day to slow down and focus on the present moment.

d. Avoid multitasking: Focus on one task at a time and give it your full attention.

By incorporating these practices into your daily routine, you can cultivate a greater sense of self-kindness, common humanity, and mindfulness, leading to greater well-being and personal growth.

Overcoming Self-compassion Barriers.

Self-compassion is the ability to be kind, supportive and understanding towards yourself, especially during times of difficulty and struggle. However, many people face common barriers to self-compassion, such as self-criticism and perfectionism, which can make it challenging to develop a more compassionate and accepting relationship with oneself. Here are some ways to overcome these barriers and cultivate self-compassion:

1. Practice self-awareness: Start by becoming more aware of your thoughts and emotions. Notice when you are being self-critical or perfectionistic, and try to understand why you feel this way. Often, negative self-talk is driven by underlying fears and beliefs that we may not even be aware of.

2. Challenge negative self-talk: When you notice negative self-talk, challenge it by asking

yourself if it is true, helpful, or kind. If it isn't, reframe the thought in a more positive and compassionate way. For example, instead of saying "I'm such an idiot for making that mistake," say "Everyone makes mistakes, and I can learn from this experience."

3. Practice self-compassion exercises: There are many exercises and techniques you can use to cultivate self-compassion, such as self-compassion meditation, writing a

self-compassion letter, or creating a self-compassion mantra. These exercises can help you to develop a more compassionate and accepting relationship with yourself.

4. Set realistic expectations: Perfectionism can be a significant barrier to self-compassion. Set realistic expectations for yourself, and acknowledge that you are human and will make mistakes. Remember that self-compassion does not mean lowering your standards, but rather being kind

and understanding when you fall short.

5. Seek support: Finally, seek support from others. Talk to friends or family members, or consider working with a therapist or coach who can help you develop self-compassion skills and overcome barriers to self-compassion.

Remember, developing self-compassion is a process that takes time and practice. Be patient with yourself and keep working towards a more compassionate and accepting relationship with yourself.

Chapter 3

Benefits of Self-Compassion.

Self-compassion is a powerful tool that can help individuals navigate common mental health challenges such as anxiety, depression, and stress in the following ways:

1. Reducing self-criticism: Self-compassion helps individuals to let go of self-judgment and self-criticism, which are common characteristics of anxiety and depression. By practicing

self-compassion, individuals can learn to be more understanding and accepting of themselves, which can help to reduce feelings of shame and guilt.

2. Building resilience: Self-compassion helps individuals to develop a stronger sense of resilience, which is the ability to bounce back from difficult situations. By being kind and supportive to oneself, individuals can develop a sense of inner strength that can help them

cope with stressors more effectively.

3. Improving emotional regulation: Self-compassion can also help individuals to regulate their emotions more effectively. By acknowledging and accepting difficult emotions, individuals can learn to be more mindful and present, which can reduce feelings of overwhelm and anxiety.

4. Promoting self-care: Practicing self-compassion also involves

taking care of oneself, which is an essential aspect of mental health. By prioritizing self-care activities, such as exercise, healthy eating, and spending time with loved ones, individuals can boost their overall well-being and resilience.

Overall, self-compassion is a powerful tool that can help individuals navigate common mental health challenges. By practicing self-compassion, individuals can reduce self-criticism, build resilience, improve emotional regulation, and promote self-care, all of which can lead to a more fulfilling and healthy life.

Self-compassion And Resilience.

Here are some ways to use self-compassion to manage difficult emotions, develop greater self-awareness, and build resilience in the face of adversity:

1. Acknowledge and validate your emotions: When we experience difficult emotions such as

sadness, anger, or anxiety, it is important to acknowledge and validate our feelings. Self-compassion involves accepting that it is natural to feel these emotions and that they are a part of the human experience.

2. Practice mindfulness: Mindfulness involves being present in the moment and observing our thoughts and feelings without judgment. When we practice mindfulness, we can become more aware of our emotions and learn to respond to

them with greater self-compassion.

3. Use positive self-talk: The way we talk to ourselves can have a big impact on our emotions and well-being. Instead of criticizing or berating ourselves, we can use positive self-talk to encourage and support ourselves. For example, we might say, "It's okay to feel upset right now. I am doing the best I can."

4. Practice self-care: Taking care of ourselves is an important aspect

of self-compassion. This might involve getting enough sleep, eating well, exercising, spending time in nature, or engaging in activities that bring us joy and fulfillment.

5. Cultivate gratitude: Gratitude involves focusing on the positive aspects of our lives and appreciating what we have. When we cultivate gratitude, we can develop a more positive outlook on life and build resilience in the face of adversity.

6. Seek support: Finally, it is important to seek support from others when we are going through difficult times. This might involve talking to a trusted friend, family member, or mental health professional. Seeking support is a sign of strength, not weakness, and can help us to build resilience and cope with difficult emotions more effectively.

Self-compassion For Relationships.

Self-compassion is an important aspect of building fulfilling and meaningful relationships with others. Here are some ways to use self-compassion to enhance your relationships:

1. Practice self-acceptance: Start by accepting yourself for who you are, including your flaws and imperfections. Recognize that everyone has their own strengths and weaknesses, and that you are

no exception. Self-acceptance will help you to build self-confidence and develop a more positive self-image.

2. Practice self-forgiveness: Everyone makes mistakes, and it's important to learn how to forgive yourself when you do. Acknowledge your mistakes, but don't dwell on them or beat yourself up about them. Instead, learn from them and move on.

3. Practice self-care: Taking care of yourself physically, emotionally,

and mentally is essential to building fulfilling relationships with others. Make sure to prioritize self-care activities such as exercise, healthy eating, getting enough sleep, and engaging in activities that bring you joy.

4. Practice empathy: Empathy involves being able to put yourself in someone else's shoes and understand their perspective. When you practice empathy, you become more understanding and accepting of others, which can

lead to deeper and more meaningful relationships.

5. Practice vulnerability: Being vulnerable means being open and honest with others about your thoughts and feelings, even if they may be uncomfortable or difficult to share. When you practice vulnerability, you allow others to get to know the real you, which can lead to more authentic and fulfilling relationships.

Overall, developing self-compassion is key to building more fulfilling and meaningful relationships with others. By practicing self-acceptance, self-forgiveness, self-care, empathy, and vulnerability, you can build stronger connections with those around you and deepen your sense of belonging and connection in the world.

Chapter 4

Self-Compassion Applications.

Self-compassion can have a wide range of practical applications in daily life. Here are a few examples:

1. Coping with difficult emotions: When you experience negative emotions like anxiety, sadness, or anger, practicing self-compassion can help you be more accepting of your feelings and provide comfort and support to yourself. You can remind yourself that it's normal

to feel this way and offer yourself kindness and understanding.

2. Overcoming self-criticism: Self-compassion can help you challenge negative self-talk and reduce self-criticism. Instead of being hard on yourself for mistakes or shortcomings, you can practice self-compassion by treating yourself with kindness and understanding, and offering yourself words of encouragement.

3. Managing stress: Self-compassion can be a

powerful tool for managing stress. When you're feeling overwhelmed or under pressure, you can offer yourself self-compassion by taking a break, engaging in a self-care activity, or reminding yourself that you're doing the best you can.

4. Improving relationships: Practicing self-compassion can also improve your relationships with others. When you're kind and understanding with yourself, you're more likely to extend that

same kindness and understanding to others. This can improve your communication, empathy, and overall relationship satisfaction.

5. Enhancing well-being: Self-compassion has been linked to greater levels of well-being, including higher levels of self-esteem, resilience, and life satisfaction. By practicing self-compassion regularly, you can enhance your overall sense of well-being and lead a happier, more fulfilling life.

Self-compassion for Boundaries

Self-compassion can help you set boundaries, make decisions, and communicate with others in a kind and respectful way by allowing you to tune in to your own needs and values without criticizing or berating yourself. Here are some steps you can take to use self-compassion in these situations:

1. Set clear boundaries based on your values and needs: Self-compassion involves recognizing and honoring your own needs and values, even if they conflict with others'. When setting boundaries, it can be helpful to first check in with yourself and identify what you need and want. Then, communicate your needs and boundaries to others in a kind and respectful way, without apologizing or justifying yourself excessively. Remember that setting boundaries is not about

controlling or manipulating others, but rather about taking care of yourself and your own well-being.

2. Make decisions based on self-compassion: Making decisions can be stressful and overwhelming, especially if you are worried about disappointing others or making mistakes. To make decisions with self-compassion, try to approach the situation with a curious and open mindset, rather than a critical or judgmental one. Allow

yourself to explore different options without rushing or pressuring yourself to make a choice. Trust that you are capable of making a good decision based on your own values and priorities.

3. Communicate with others in a kind and respectful way: Communicating with others can be challenging, especially if you are feeling upset or frustrated. To communicate with self-compassion, try to first acknowledge and validate your

own feelings, without blaming or criticizing yourself or others. Then, approach the conversation with a willingness to listen and understand the other person's perspective, rather than assuming the worst or getting defensive. Remember that everyone is doing the best they can with the resources they have, and that you can choose to respond in a kind and respectful way, even if you disagree with the other person's behavior or opinion.

Overall, using self-compassion to set boundaries, make decisions, and communicate with others involves treating yourself and others with kindness, understanding, and respect, even in difficult situations. It takes practice and patience, but can lead to greater self-awareness, confidence, and well-being in the long run.

Self-compassion for self-care.

It involves acknowledging your struggles and shortcomings without judgment and with a desire to learn and grow. By cultivating self-compassion, you can develop a more positive and empowering relationship with yourself, which can lead to greater self-care and well-being. Here are some ways to use self-compassion to cultivate greater self-care:

1. Practice mindfulness: Mindfulness can help you become more aware of your thoughts and emotions, and help you observe them without judgment. This can help you identify negative

self-talk and respond to it with self-compassion.

2. Treat yourself like you would treat a friend: Imagine that a friend was going through a difficult time. You would likely offer them words of support, understanding, and kindness. Try treating yourself with the same level of care and compassion.

3. Reframe negative self-talk: When you catch yourself engaging in negative self-talk, try reframing it in a more positive light. For

example, instead of saying "I'm so stupid for making that mistake," say "I made a mistake, but I can learn from it and do better next time."

4. Practice self-care: Engage in activities that nourish your mind, body, and spirit, such as exercise, eating healthy, getting enough sleep, and practicing self-care routines.

5. Forgive yourself: It's important to acknowledge that everyone makes mistakes, and it's okay to

forgive yourself for them. Instead of dwelling on past mistakes, try to learn from them and move forward with self-compassion.

6. Practice gratitude: Take time each day to reflect on the things in your life that you are grateful for. This can help shift your focus away from negative self-talk and cultivate a more positive mindset.

Remember, cultivating self-compassion takes time and practice. Be patient and kind to yourself as you develop this important skill.

Chapter 5

Self-compassion's Transformative Power.

Instead of being self-critical or judgmental, self-compassion involves cultivating a non-judgmental awareness of one's own thoughts and feelings, and responding with warmth and empathy.

The transformative power of self-compassion lies in its ability to foster resilience, emotional well-being, and personal growth. By treating ourselves with kindness and compassion, we can learn to manage difficult emotions and overcome setbacks with greater ease. This can help us to avoid getting stuck in negative thought patterns, and to bounce back from adversity more quickly.

Research has shown that self-compassion is associated with greater life satisfaction, lower levels of anxiety and depression, and higher levels of motivation and self-esteem. People who practice self-compassion are also more likely to engage in healthy behaviors, such as exercise and self-care, and to have more positive social relationships.

Self-compassion can be cultivated through various practices, such as mindfulness meditation, writing self-compassionate letters to oneself, and practicing self-compassion in daily life. These practices involve developing a non-judgmental awareness of one's own thoughts and feelings, and learning to respond to oneself with kindness and understanding.

Self-compassion integration.

Integrating self-compassion into your daily routine can help you develop a more compassionate and accepting relationship with yourself. Here are some tips on how to do it:

1. Practice mindfulness: Mindfulness can help you become more aware of your thoughts, feelings, and physical sensations. When you notice negative self-talk, try to acknowledge it

and replace it with kinder, more supportive words.

2. Treat yourself like you would treat a friend: If a friend was going through a tough time, you would likely be compassionate and supportive. Try to treat yourself with the same kindness and understanding.

3. Take care of your physical needs: Make sure you're getting enough sleep, eating well, and getting enough exercise. Taking care of your physical needs can help you

feel better emotionally, which can make it easier to be compassionate toward yourself.

4. Celebrate your accomplishments: Take time to recognize and celebrate your achievements, no matter how small they may be. Acknowledging your accomplishments can help you build self-confidence and self-esteem.

5. Practice self-acceptance: Accepting yourself for who you are, flaws and all, can be a

powerful act of self-compassion. Remember that everyone makes mistakes, and that you are worthy of love and respect just as you are.

6. Seek support: Sometimes, it can be difficult to be compassionate toward ourselves on our own. If you're struggling, don't hesitate to reach out to a therapist or a trusted friend for support.

Self-compassion for Resilience

Cultivating self-compassion can have a significant impact on one's resilience and ability to navigate the challenges of life with greater ease and grace. Here are some ways in which self-compassion can help:

1. Reduced self-criticism: When we face a setback or failure, we often engage in self-criticism, which can be harsh and unproductive. Self-compassion involves recognizing that failure and setbacks are a part of life and treating oneself with kindness

and understanding. This approach can help reduce self-criticism and increase self-acceptance, which can be beneficial in building resilience.

2. Greater emotional regulation: Self-compassion can help us regulate our emotions more effectively by reducing the intensity and duration of negative emotions. When we are kind to ourselves, we are less likely to engage in negative self-talk or rumination, which can exacerbate negative emotions.

3. Improved coping strategies: When we approach difficult situations with self-compassion, we are more likely to engage in adaptive coping strategies, such as seeking social support, problem-solving, and positive reframing. These strategies can help us navigate challenging situations more effectively and increase our resilience.

4. Increased self-care: Self-compassion involves taking care of oneself in a kind and

nurturing way. This can involve engaging in activities that promote physical and emotional well-being, such as exercise, meditation, and spending time with loved ones. Taking care of oneself can improve overall resilience and help us navigate the ups and downs of life more effectively.

Conclusion

In this book, we have explored the power of self-compassion, and how it can help you navigate mental health challenges with grace and resilience. Through the practical strategies and exercises outlined in this book, you can develop a more compassionate and accepting relationship with yourself, and cultivate greater well-being and happiness in your daily life. Remember, self-compassion is a powerful tool that can help you navigate life's challenges with greater ease and grace, and it is always within your reach.

www.ingramcontent.com/pod-product-compliance
Lightning Source LLC
Chambersburg PA
CBHW071034220526
45467CB00004B/1656